Alternative Treatments of Insomnia

Safe, effective and affordable approaches and how to use them

James Lake, MD

This book is dedicated to my best friend and soul mate, Nicole Asselborn, MD, with gratitude for invaluable advice on the right scope and 'voice' for this project, and for creating the lovely image on the cover.

Contents

Part I: Introduction

- What this book is about
- How to use this book
- Alternative and integrative medicine defined
- Integrative mental health care defined
- About Dr. Lake's background and qualifications
- What to do if you have severe insomnia

Part II: Understanding and treating insomnia from a holistic point of view

- Understanding insomnia
- Taking inventory
- Identifying treatments that make sense for you: evaluating the evidence
- Alternative treatments of insomnia
- Deciding on a treatment plan that is *right for you*
- Making changes along the way: re-evaluating your treatment plan and making it better
- Repeating the steps until you find a treatment plan that works *for you*

- Summary of main points

Going deeper

Finding quality products and services on the internet

Disclaimer

The information provided in this book is intended to provide helpful information on the treatment of insomnia and does not constitute medical advice. The publisher and author are not responsible for any specific health needs that may require medical supervision and are not liable for any damages or negative consequences from any treatment, action or application to any person reading or using the information in this book. References to internet resources are provided for informational purposes only and do not constitute endorsement of any websites or other sources. Readers should be aware that the websites listed in this book may change.

Part I: Introduction

What this book is about

My chief goal in writing this book and the others in the series was to create a practical low-cost resource on safe and effective alternative treatments of mental health problems including herbals, vitamins and other natural supplements, mind-body approaches, and energy therapies.

The subject of this book is insomnia. You will learn about a variety of safe and effective alternative treatments of insomnia. If you have chronic insomnia, you are taking a medication that isn't helping, experiencing side effects, or you can't afford to continue taking a medication that *is working* this book provides valuable information about a variety of alternative treatments of insomnia and practical strategies for how to use them.

If you've had insomnia in the past and you are sleeping consistently better now this book will help you create a wellness plan that fits your lifestyle and your budget. By the time you finish reading you'll be able to create an individualized care plan adapted to your needs, preferences and budget. Just as important, you will learn how to *think about* your mental health in a more holistic way.

How to use this book

This book was *written to give you the maximum amount of information in the least amount of time*. The last section of the book is a summary of the most important points. I've provided links to valuable internet resources to help you find quality brands of natural supplements and other alternative treatments, important safety information and professional help if you think you need it.

If you are a mental healthcare professional this book provides concise, jargon-free summaries of scientifically validated alternative treatments you can use when advising clients about safe and effective alternative treatments of insomnia.

Alternative and integrative medicine defined

Alternative medicine—sometimes called 'complementary and alternative medicine or CAM—consists of approaches that are currently not used in mainstream Western medicine (also called 'biomedicine' and 'allopathic medicine'). Examples of CAM include acupuncture, herbs and other natural supplements, so-called 'energy' therapies such as Healing Touch, and others.

Integrative medicine is a rapidly growing model of care that takes a middle ground between Western medicine as conventionally practiced and CAM. Integrative medicine:

- is a person-centered approach

- that takes account of the needs and preferences of each unique person

- that focuses on maintaining optimal health and treating symptoms

- uses both conventional mainstream approaches like medications and psychotherapy, and complementary and alternative (CAM) therapies like herbal medicines and acupuncture

- is based on the *best available* scientific evidence

Integrative mental health care defined

Integrative mental health care is a specialized area of integrative medicine aimed at helping each person find safe, appropriate and effective treatments for their mental health problem taking into account their unique symptoms, values, preferences and circumstances.

Integrative mental health care often includes advice on life-style changes that require on-going commitment to improving health and mental health such as changing your diet, exercising more, sleeping better, and using relaxation techniques to reduce stress. In addition to lifestyle changes integrative mental health care may include advice on select herbals, vitamins and other natural supplements when there is evidence for both their safety and effectiveness. Finally, Integrative mental health care may include medications or other conventionally used treatments.

If this is the first time you've heard about integrative mental health care and want to find out more before trying a new treatment for insomnia, I encourage you to download the first book in the series to learn more. The book is available as a free download and will give you an overview of essential concepts and methods in integrative mental health care.

About Dr. Lake's background and qualifications

I completed my medical training at University of California, Irvine, and did my residency in adult psychiatry at Stanford University Hospital. I am board-certified by the American Board of Psychiatry and Neurology, and I have practiced psychiatry for more than 20 years in diverse settings. I've had extensive experience taking care of patients in hospitals, clinics, emergency rooms and in my private practice. I have been a student of herbal medicine for decades and I am certified in medical acupuncture and in EEG biofeedback. I previously served on the teaching faculty at Stanford University Hospital and I am currently an adjunct clinical assistant professor in the Department of Psychiatry at University of Arizona College of Medicine. I've taught physicians and other mental health professionals about integrative mental healthcare at national and international conferences. I publish a column on integrative mental health care in *Psychiatric Times,* a leading trade publication for mental health professionals and I am a frequent blogger on Psychology Today. I've authored numerous articles and chapters in medical journals and textbooks, and I've written, co-authored or edited five textbooks covering the philosophy, theory and practice of integrative mental healthcare.

I've been involved in national and international efforts to establish integrative mental healthcare as a new medical sub-specialty in its own right. I founded and previously chaired an initiative aimed at changing mental health care into a more effective, safer and more person-centered model of care: the American Psychiatric Association Caucus on Complementary and Integrative Medicine. An important goal of the Caucus is the development of expert resources for educating and training psychiatrists in the safe, *evidence-based* uses of non-medication treatments for treating anxiety, depression and the other common mental health problems covered in the book series.

What to do if you have severe insomnia

Severe symptoms of insomnia include:

- Difficulty falling asleep almost every night without taking a sleep aid

- Experiencing frequent awakenings throughout the night

- Waking up early and being unable to return to sleep

- Recurring disturbing dreams or nightmares

- Frequent 'automatic behaviors' when sleeping such as sleep walking or involuntary leg movements

Insomnia is severe when it lasts for weeks or longer and results in considerable distress, extreme fatigue, or symptoms of cognitive impairment that interfere with one's capacity to function at work, in school, or in other day to day activities.

If you have severe insomnia you may need more help than this book can provide. For example, you may need to take a sedative on a regular basis in order to sleep consistently well. Even if you need to take a prescription sleep aid, you may benefit from the approaches described in this book. *If in addition to insomnia you are severely depressed or have another serious mental health problem, I encourage you to seek urgent care from a psychiatrist or other mental healthcare provider.*

Part II: Understanding and treating insomnia from an integrative point of view

The information in the following sections will help you to better understand your sleep problem and will give you the tools you need to develop a safe, effective and affordable treatment plan.

Understanding insomnia

Nighttime sleep and daytime wakefulness are regulated by many neurotransmitters including the brain's principle inhibitory neurotransmitter gamma-aminobutyric acid (GABA). Changing brain levels of GABA and other neurotransmitters are believed to be related to normal changes in sleep with healthy aging.

What constitutes *normal* sleep varies considerably between different cultures and demographic groups. For example, healthy elderly individuals sleep less at night compared to young and middle-aged individuals and make up for reduced night-time sleep by spending more time napping during the day.

It is estimated that chronic insomnia affects at least one third of the world's population. Nighttime insomnia and daytime sleepiness are major public health issues because they result in enormous losses in work productivity and significantly increase the risk of workplace and motor vehicle accidents.

A variety of medical and mental health problems interfere with one's ability to fall asleep, sleep without interruption through the night, or achieve restful sleep. Diverse social, cultural, psychological and biological factors affect sleep and most cases of insomnia are caused by a variety of factors. Approximately two thirds of individuals treated for any mental health problem complain of chronic insomnia. Individuals who struggle with chronic depressed mood or anxiety or who abuse alcohol or drugs are especially at risk for insomnia. Depending on the drug of abuse, insomnia may be a direct result of substance use or a symptom of withdrawal when a person abruptly stops drinking or using a drug following a prolonged period of abuse.

Insomnia is a core symptom of bipolar mania and post-traumatic stress disorder (PTSD). Insomnia frequently accompanies medical problems such as chronic pain, sleep apnea, diabetes, lung diseases, thyroid disease, dementia and neurological disorders. Sleep apnea is a medical condition in which difficulty breathing during sleep causes frequent waking throughout the night resulting in severe daytime sleepiness. Sleep apnea is associated with a significantly increased risk of depressed mood, overweight and heart disease. Elderly persons who have serious medical or mental health problems are especially at risk of chronic insomnia.

Insomnia is a frequently reported side effect of many medications including antidepressants and other psychotropic medications. Individuals who do shift-work (i.e. whose work schedule begins late night and continues until early morning) or travel extensively across many time-zones often experience insomnia related to a disturbance in their biological clock. Sleep disorders related to shift work and frequent international travel are called *circadian rhythm sleep disorders*. Some individuals experience disrupted sleep because of recurring nightmares or so-called *sleep automatisms* such as sleep walking, or abnormal leg movements that typically occur during the deepest stages of sleep (i.e., rapid-eye movement or REM sleep).

On the opposite extreme from chronic insomnia, some individuals complain of excessive sleep (i.e., compared to sleep requirements of the average person within their culture or demographic group) but may nevertheless experience severe symptoms of daytime fatigue and sleepiness.

Taking inventory of your symptoms

This section will help you understand your sleeping problem and determine how severe it is. Let's start by defining what the word *symptom* means. A *symptom is something you experience inside that you can't see. It's a subjective experience of distress that can point to an underlying medical or mental health problem.* When different symptoms occur together, they make up a particular mental health problem or *disorder*.

While many individuals who struggle with insomnia have similar symptoms, each person's symptoms are related to their *unique* genetic and biological constitution, social and family history, cultural and spiritual beliefs, and personal circumstances. Symptoms of insomnia can be mild, moderate or severe depending on how much distress they cause and how much they interfere with your ability to function in day to day activities.

Taking inventory of your symptoms of insomnia involves filling in a check-list or answering standardized questions. Going through this process will give you important insights that will help you put together a treatment plan based on your particular symptoms. If you are reading the e-book you can click here to get to psychological assessment tools that you can use to evaluate your sleep problem and the other mental health problems covered in this series of books. If you are reading the print book you can find on-line psychological assessment tools at http://www.theintegrativementalhealthsolution.com/self-assesment-questionaires.html.

Remember to keep a record of your results so that you can track changes in your symptoms over time. It is a good idea to take inventory frequently in order to find out how well your symptoms of insomnia are responding to treatment. You can use the results to optimize your current treatment plan or develop a completely new treatment plan.

If you have severe insomnia together with another mental health problem, I encourage you to complete the self-assessment inventory for that problem also.

Identifying treatments that make sense for you: evaluating the evidence

This section provides concise reviews of the evidence for a variety of alternative treatments of insomnia. In addition to natural supplements and prescription medications, other approaches that are beneficial for insomnia include EEG biofeedback therapy, early morning bright light exposure therapy, acupuncture, mindfulness-based stress reduction (MBSR), micro-current electrical stimulation and yoga.

Natural supplements used to treat insomnia include melatonin, the amino acids L-tryptophan, 5-hydroxytryptophan, and the herbals *Withania somnifera* (Ashwagandha), Ginseng (*Panax ginseng*), *Ginkgo biloba*, and St. John's wort (*Hypericum perforatum*). Most herbals and other natural supplements have few or mild side effects when a quality brand is used at the recommended dosage. However, some natural supplements can cause potentially serious side effects when taken at inappropriate high dosages or in combination with certain medications. *Please read the comments on safety before trying any herbal or other natural supplement.*

The various alternative approaches used to treat insomnia can be divided into 5 categories:

- **Biological treatments** have beneficial effects at the level of one or more well-defined molecular mechanism. Natural supplements work in this way.

- **Whole body approaches** have general beneficial effects on the body as a whole, improve both physical and mental health and enhance well-being. Exercise and massage are examples of whole-body approaches.

- **Mindfulness and mind-body approaches** are based on concepts from traditional healing aimed at improving the harmony between mind and body. Approaches in this category include awareness training, breathing techniques and mental imagery. While some mindfulness and mind-body approaches are based on a particular spiritual belief system, you do not need to believe in God or have a spiritual orientation in order to benefit from these practices. Yoga, Tai-chi, and transcendental meditation are examples.

- **Treatments based on scientifically verified forms of energy** including electricity, magnetic fields, light and sound have beneficial effects at many levels in the body and brain. Examples include full-spectrum bright light exposure, weak electrical current, EEG biofeedback, and specialized forms of sound therapy.

- **Treatments based on 'subtle' forms of energy** that have not been verified by science such as Reiki, qigong, prayer, Healing Touch and Therapeutic Touch may be beneficial at the level of postulated energetic processes that may play a role in maintaining optimal physical and psychological wellness, and for treating some mental health problems.

Most vitamins, minerals and essential fatty acids are examples of natural supplements that can be safely used without the advice or supervision of a physician or other health care provider. However, some natural supplements derived from plants or other natural products cause potentially serious safety problems and it is important to adhere to recommended dosages when using these supplements and avoid taking them with medications known to cause unsafe toxic interactions.

When a natural supplement is associated with potentially serious adverse effects or toxicities ***important safety warnings are in bold face, underlined and in italics***. ***I encourage you to consult with a knowledgeable health care provider for advice on the safe and appropriate use of any supplement that has potentially serious adverse effects***.

While some people prefer to use a medication or a natural supplement only, others benefit from combining a supplement or medication with a mind-body practice, acupuncture or another approach. The treatment plan you ultimately decide on will depend not only on the scientific evidence supporting it, but also the amount of time you have to try a particular approach, and your level of motivation.

While there are no potential safety problems associated with approaches such as EEG biofeedback and acupuncture, it may take a great deal of time, effort and training to benefit from such therapies.

Finally, you may have a better or more rapid response if you consistently try an approach such as exercise, yoga or another mind-body practice while taking an appropriate supplement or a medication. Such combined treatment regimens are examples of integrative mental health care, as described above.

Alternative treatments of insomnia

This section reviews the evidence for specific herbals and other natural products, exercise, mind-body approaches, and energy therapies such as bright light exposure therapy and EEG biofeedback. The information under each modality is listed in bullets so that you can compare research evidence and safety information for a variety of treatment choices:

- Name of treatment and category

- How the treatment works (where known)

- Dosages (for natural supplements) or frequency or duration of use (for whole body, mind-body or energy approaches)

- Examples of safe and effective treatment combinations

- Comments about adverse effects and warnings pertaining to the treatment or treatment combination that may result in potentially unsafe interactions and should be avoided

- Average duration of treatment needed to achieve beneficial results

I use a 3-tier approach to rate treatments based on the relative strength of evidence.

- **Tier A:** treatments are supported by strong research evidence from rigorously conducted studies or systematic reviews of studies.

- **Tier B:** treatments are also supported by research evidence but not to the same degree as tier A treatments.

- **Tier C:** treatments are supported by weak or inconsistent research findings and may be effective in some cases

Note that treatments under each tier are listed in alphabetical order and not according to the relative level of evidence.

Tier A treatments of insomnia

- <u>EEG biofeedback training</u>

- <u>Bright light exposure therapy</u>

- <u>Valerian (*Valeriana officinalis*)</u>

EEG biofeedback training (Also called *neuro-feedback* and *neural therapy*)

- **Name of treatment and category:** EEG biofeedback training is a scientifically validated energy therapy.

- **How the treatment works:** EEG biofeedback training decreases the severity of chronic insomnia by changing electrical activity in brain regions involved in regulating sleep and wakefulness including the sensory motor cortex and other areas. Insomnia is often associated with problems thinking during the daytime. Some individuals who achieve improved sleep with EEG biofeedback training experience generally improved cognitive functioning.

- **Dosages (for natural supplements) or frequency of use (for whole body, mind-body or energy approaches):** A specialized EEG biofeedback training program consisting of 10 to 15, 20 minute sessions administered weekly or more often can significantly improve the duration and quality of sleep in individuals with chronic insomnia.

- **Examples of safe and effective treatment combinations: EEG biofeedback may be safely used in combination with other treatments of insomnia.** Regular EEG biofeedback training for individuals with chronic insomnia permits some individuals to reduce their dosage of prescription sleep medications.

- **Comments about adverse effects and warnings pertaining to treatment combinations that may result in potentially unsafe interactions and should be avoided:** Some individuals experience mild transient dizziness or headache following EEG biofeedback training.

- **Average duration of treatment needed to achieve beneficial results:** Some individuals experience sustained improvement in sleep quality and duration after 1 to 2 weeks of daily EEG biofeedback training.

Bright light exposure therapy

- **Name of treatment and category:** Bright light exposure is a scientifically validated energy treatment.

- **How the treatment works:** Light exposure therapy affects the timing of melatonin secretion in the brain. Some individuals who have chronic insomnia due to shift work or jet lag have confused sleep-wake cycles. In such cases early morning exposure to full-spectrum bright light decreases the level of melatonin secreted in the brain, increases daytime wakefulness and resets the timing of melatonin secretion returning the sleep-wake cycle to its normal pattern and improving sleep quality. Early morning bright light exposure may also decrease symptoms of depressed mood which often occur together with chronic insomnia.

- **Dosages (for natural supplements) or frequency of use (for whole body, mind-body or energy approaches):** Many individuals who experience insomnia related to jet lag or shift work benefit from daily early morning bright light (approximately 10,000 lux) exposure lasting 30 to 40 minutes. Orienting toward the early morning sunlight (i.e. if there is bright sunshine) with the eyes closed is as effective as using an artificial light source. *NOTE: The timing of bright light exposure is very important and bright light exposure in the late morning or afternoon may have no effect on sleep or may worsen insomnia.*

- **Examples of safe and effective treatment combinations:** Taking melatonin soon before bedtime may increase the beneficial effects of early morning bright light exposure and result in more rapid improvement in insomnia. Consuming foods rich in L-tryptophan such as meats, eggs, grains and milk especially for breakfast, may have beneficial additive effects to early morning bright light exposure for the treatment of insomnia.

- **Comments about adverse effects and warnings pertaining to treatment combinations that may result in potentially unsafe interactions and should be avoided:** Bright light exposure is generally safe when practiced according to suggested guidelines. *Caution: Early morning bright light exposure may cause hypomania in individuals diagnosed with bipolar disorder. Caution: Never stare directly at the sum as it can cause permanent eye damage or blindness. Caution: If you use an artificial light source be sure to use* _only lights that do not emit ultraviolet light (which can_

cause permanent eye damage or blindness).

- **Average duration of treatment needed to achieve beneficial results:** Daily early morning bright light exposure can re-set the sleep-wake cycle and improve symptoms of insomnia after several days.

Valerian (_Valeriana officinalis_)

- **Name of treatment and category:** _Valeriana officinalis_ is an herbal medicine used to treat insomnia and stress.

- **How the treatment:** The active ingredients of _V. officinalis_ affect neurotransmitters in the brain causing mild sedation.

- **Dosages (for natural supplements) or frequency of use (for whole body, mind-body or energy approaches):** A standardized extract of _V. officinalis_ taken at a dose of 600mg to 900mg at bedtime improves the quality and duration of sleep. _V. officinalis_ may be as effective as some prescription sleep aids for the treatment of chronic insomnia.

- **Examples of safe and effective treatment combinations:** It is preferable to avoid taking *V. officinalis* in combination with other natural products or prescription medications (see below).

- **Comments about adverse effects and warnings pertaining to treatment combinations that may result in potentially unsafe interactions and should be avoided:** *V. officinalis* is safe with few mild adverse effects when a standardized preparation is taken following suggested dosage guidelines. *Caution: V. officinalis should not be used in combination with prescription sleep medications or alcohol as this may result in severe sedation. Caution: V. officinalis taken in large doses may cause elevation in liver enzymes. Warning: some active ingredients of V. officinalis may* _**cause birth defects and should be avoided in women who are pregnant or nursing.**_

- **Average duration of treatment needed to achieve beneficial results:** Many individuals experience sustained improvement in the quality and duration of sleep after taking the recommended dosage of a standardized preparation of _V. officinalis_ for 2 to 6 weeks.

Tier B treatments of insomnia

- Acupuncture

- Cranial electrotherapy stimulation (CES)

- Exercise

- L-tryptophan and 5-hydroxytryptophan (5-HTP)

- Melatonin

- Mindfulness-based Stress Reduction (MBSR)

- <u>Music</u>

Acupuncture

- **Name of treatment and category:** Acupuncture is an energy technique used in traditional Asian healing in which fine needles are inserted at specific points on the body.

- **How the treatment works:** Beneficial effects of acupuncture are probably related to several different mechanisms. Acupuncture protocols that improve sleep are believed to release endorphins or other neurotransmitters that have general calming effects on the brain. Many types of acupuncture exist including conventional manual acupuncture, electro-acupuncture and laser acupuncture. A specialized kind of acupuncture called ariculo-therapy (i.e. ear acupuncture) involves the insertion of magnetic pellets on the ears.

- **Dosages (for natural supplements) or frequency of use (for whole body, mind-body or energy approaches):** Typical acupuncture treatment sessions may last 20 to 30 minutes or longer. The specific acupuncture points stimulated, the acupuncture technique used and intervals between treatments are determined by assessment findings that point to an energetic imbalance manifesting as insomnia. Ear acupuncture using magnetic pearls (but not needles) may improve the quality and duration of sleep in individuals with chronic insomnia. Acupuncture is an effective and safe treatment of depressed mood, anxiety and other mental health problems that often occur together with chronic insomnia.

- **Examples of safe and effective treatment combinations:** Acupuncture may be safely used in combination with prescription medications, natural products or other approaches.

- **Comments about adverse effects and warnings pertaining to treatment combinations that may result in potentially unsafe interactions and should be avoided:** Acupuncture is generally safe when practiced according to established guidelines however there are rare reports of infection and bleeding.

- **Average duration of treatment needed to achieve beneficial results:** Some individuals with chronic insomnia experience improvements in sleep that may last for months following 2 to 3 weeks of regular acupuncture treatment.

Cranial electrotherapy stimulation (CES)

- **Name of treatment and category:** CES is a scientifically validated energy therapy.

- **How the treatment works:** In CES a weak electrical current is applied to the head or earlobes with the goal changing brain electrical activity or neurotransmitters resulting in improved sleep. Regular CES therapy may reduce the amount of time needed for some individuals to fall asleep and increase total sleep duration. Regular CES therapy may decrease symptoms of generalized anxiety and moderate cognitive problems in individuals in the early stages of dementia, who often have disturbed sleep. Insomnia is a common problem in anxious and demented individuals.

- **Dosages (for natural supplements) or frequency of use (for whole body, mind-body or energy approaches):** The optimal frequency, amperage and waveform of electrical current employed in CES may vary depending on the severity of insomnia. CES treatments for insomnia are often administered as a series of daily 60 minutes sessions.

- **Examples of safe and effective treatment combinations:** CES may be safely used in combination with a prescription medication, a natural supplement, or other complementary and alternative treatments of insomnia. Some individuals experience greater improvement in sleep with CES treatments alone compared to CES plus a prescription sleep aid.

- **Comments about adverse effects and warnings pertaining to treatment combinations that may result in potentially unsafe interactions and should be avoided:** CES is generally safe when administered according to suggested guidelines. Some individuals experience mild tingling sensations during treatment. *__Caution: CES may cause an abnormal heart rhythm and should not be used by anyone with a cardiac pacemaker.__*

- **Average duration of treatment needed to achieve beneficial results:** For best results CES should be used daily for several weeks. Some individuals with chronic insomnia experience sustained improvements in the quality and duration of sleep after a series of 3 to 5 daily CES treatments lasting 60 minutes.

Exercise

- **Name of treatment and category:** Exercise is a whole-body approach.

- **How the treatment works:** Regular exercise such as walking, cycling, running and weight lifting reduces stress, enhances general well-being and improves sleep quality and duration. Regular exercise decreases the severity of depressed mood and anxiety which frequently occur together with insomnia.

- **Dosages (for natural supplements) or frequency of use (for whole body, mind-body or energy approaches):** Regular exercise 2 to 3 times weekly lasting at least 30 minutes may improve sleep quality and general health and well-being.

- **Examples of safe and effective treatment combinations:** Physical activity and exercise can be safely combined with all other approaches.

- **Comments about adverse effects and warnings pertaining to treatment combinations that may result in potentially**

unsafe interactions and should be avoided: Engaging in regular exercise of moderate intensity is generally safe. *Caution: individuals who have heart problems, chronic pain or other serious health problems should get advice from a qualified health care provider before starting an exercise program.*

- **Average duration of treatment needed to achieve beneficial results:** Individuals who engage in regular exercise of moderate intensity at least 2 or 3 times weekly may experience significant improvements in the quality of sleep.

L-tryptophan and 5-Hydroxytryptophan (5-HTP)

- **Name of treatment and category:** L-tryptophan and 5-HTP are closely related amino acids that occur naturally in some foods and are used to treat different medical and mental health problems.

- **How the treatment works:** L-tryptophan and 5-HTP are the building blocks of neurotransmitters (e.g. melatonin and serotonin) involved in normal brain function and regulation of sleep, attention and mood.

- **Dosages (for natural supplements) or frequency of use (for whole body, mind-body or energy approaches):** There is no agreement on a standard dosage of L-tryptophan or 5-HTP for insomnia. Taking L-tryptophan at doses up to 15gm, or taking 5-HTP at doses up to 300mg just before bedtime often decreases the severity of insomnia. The effective dose of 5-HTP for insomnia is much lower than L-tryptophan because 5-HTP more readily enters the brain than L-tryptophan and is one step closer to being used as a building block of serotonin.

- **Examples of safe and effective treatment combinations:** Many individuals with chronic insomnia are depressed. L-tryptophan taken at doses up to 2gm, or 5-HTP taken at doses up to 300mg may be safely combined with a sedating antidepressant taken at bedtime. This combination may improve sleep quality and speed up the response to the antidepressant.

- **Comments about adverse effects and warnings pertaining to treatment combinations that may result in potentially unsafe interactions and should be avoided:** L-tryptophan and 5-HTP are generally safe when taken at suggested dosages and have few minor adverse effects including dizziness, drowsiness and decreased appetite. *__Caution: L-tryptophan and 5-HTP interact with some medications. It is advisable to consult with a physician or pharmacist before considering taking either substance. Note: Over two decades ago there were major safety concerns about the toxicity of L-tryptophan. Those concerns soon resolved when the apparent toxic effects of L-tryptophan were traced to a single contaminated batch.__*

- **Average duration of treatment needed to achieve beneficial results:** Many individuals with chronic insomnia experience rapid improvement in sleep after taking L-tryptophan or 5-HTP nightly for several days following suggested dosing guidelines.

Melatonin

- **Name of treatment and category:** Melatonin is a hormone that occurs naturally in the brain and is a scientifically validated treatment of insomnia.

- **How the treatment works:** Melatonin is secreted from the Pineal gland in the brain and regulates the sleep-wake cycle. Taking extra melatonin in addition to what the brain naturally produces may improve sleep quality and duration especially in individuals who have sleep problems related to shift work or jet lag. Melatonin is closely related to the neurotransmitter serotonin which plays a central role in mood regulation.

- **Dosages (for natural supplements) or frequency of use (for whole body, mind-body or energy approaches):** Taking melatonin 0.3 to 6mg soon before bedtime improves the quality of sleep. Immediate-release melatonin decreases the time needed to fall asleep. Sustained-release preparations of melatonin increase the total amount of time spent sleeping.

- **Examples of safe and effective treatment combinations:** Controlled-release melatonin (e.g. 2mg) may be safely combined with prescription sleep aids, is more effective than either approach alone and in some cases may permit a reduction in the dose of a prescription sleep aid. Early morning bright light exposure therapy can be safely used in combination with melatonin (i.e. taken before bedtime) for insomnia related to jet lag or shift work.

- **Comments about adverse effects and warnings pertaining to treatment combinations that may result in potentially**

unsafe interactions and should be avoided: Melatonin used according to suggested guidelines is generally safe with few mild adverse effects including itching, headaches, nausea and dizziness. Low doses (0.3mg) of melatonin cause no adverse effects. Some individuals who take melatonin at doses of 3mg or higher experience mild grogginess or a low body temperature the following day. Melatonin taken in the daytime may interfere with clear thinking and slow down reaction time and should be taken just before one's normal sleep schedule begins.

- **Average duration of treatment needed to achieve beneficial results:** Individuals who take melatonin often experience rapid improvement in insomnia after finding the right dose and form (i.e. immediate versus delayed release) for their particular sleep problem.

Mindfulness-based stress reduction (MBSR)

- **Name of treatment and category:** MBSR is a mindfulness practice that employs cognitive therapy techniques.

- **How the treatment works:** The regular practice of MBSR has general calming effects on the nervous system that may decrease the severity of chronic insomnia.

- **Dosages (for natural supplements) or frequency of use (for whole body, mind-body or energy approaches):** MBSR directed at improving sleep quality should ideally be practiced 30 to 45 minutes daily. Many individuals benefit from participating in a weekly MBSR group in addition to their individual mindfulness practice. The regular practice of MBSR may be as effective as prescription sleep aids for managing symptoms of chronic insomnia.

- **Examples of safe and effective treatment combinations:** MBSR may be safely used in combination with other approaches. Some individuals who engage in a regular MBSR practice or other mindfulness practice are able to decrease the dosage of prescription sleep medications without experiencing worsening in insomnia.

- **Comments about adverse effects and warnings pertaining to treatment combinations that may result in potentially unsafe interactions and should be avoided:** none

- **Average duration of treatment needed to achieve beneficial results:** The regular practice of MBSR over a period of several weeks or longer may result in sustained improvement in the severity of chronic insomnia.

Music (also called music assisted relaxation)

- **Name of treatment and category:** The use of soothing music to enhance relaxation is a scientifically validated energy healing approach.

- **How the treatment works:** Listening to calming music reduces the brain's state of arousal resulting in improved sleep.

- **Dosages (for natural supplements) or frequency of use (for whole body, mind-body or energy approaches):** The optimal type of music and the amount of time spent listening to music for the purpose of improving sleep quality have not been established. Many individuals benefit from a nightly routine of listening to soothing music for 20 to 45 minutes soon before bedtime.

- **Examples of safe and effective treatment combinations:** Music-assisted relaxation may be safely combined with other approaches.

- **Comments about adverse effects and warnings pertaining to treatment combinations that may result in potentially unsafe interactions and should be avoided:** none

- **Average duration of treatment needed to achieve beneficial results:** Many individuals with chronic insomnia experience moderate improvement in sleep quality after 1 to 2 weeks of listening to soothing music before bedtime.

Tier C treatments of insomnia

- <u>Dietary changes</u>

- <u>Herbal medicines</u>

- <u>Homeopathy</u>

- <u>Lucid dreaming training</u>

- <u>Passive body heating</u>

- <u>Relaxation techniques</u>

- <u>Yoga</u>

Dietary changes

- **Name of treatment and category:** Changes in the diet are biological treatment approaches.

- **How the treatment works:** Consuming foods rich in L-tryptophan such as meat, eggs, milk and grains, may increase nighttime melatonin secretion and improve sleep quality. Following a healthy diet consisting of vegetables, complex carbohydrates and lean meat makes it easier to fall asleep at night and sleep through the night without waking. Too little protein in the diet makes it harder to fall asleep. Too few carbohydrates in the diet makes it harder to sleep through the night. Reducing the amount of alcohol and caffeine in the diet improves the duration and quality of sleep. Drinking alcohol soon before bedtime should be avoided because it can cause you to wake up in the middle of the night. Limiting the amount of refined sugar in the diet may promote improved sleep by reducing the risk of hypoglycemia which can also cause waking during the night. Following a healthy diet helps you maintain a healthy weight and decreases the risk of developing sleep disorders related to obesity.

- **Dosages (for natural supplements) or frequency of use (for whole body, mind-body or energy approaches):** Limiting intake of caffeinated beverages to 1 to 2 servings per day and avoiding caffeine starting in the early afternoon hours may significantly reduce the risk of insomnia. Moderate alcohol consumption no later than dinnertime reduces the risk of waking up in the middle of the night.

- **Examples of safe and effective treatment combinations:** Dietary changes may be safely undertaken in combination with most prescription medications and natural supplements. However certain foods may interfere with the metabolism of some medications (below).

- **Comments about adverse effects and warnings pertaining to treatment combinations that may result in potentially unsafe interactions and should be avoided:** There are no safety concerns when following dietary changes that promote improved sleep. *__Caution: it is always advisable to consult with a qualified health care provider or pharmacist for questions or concerns about potentially unsafe__* _interactions between specific foods and medications or natural supplements._

- **Average duration of treatment needed to achieve beneficial results:** For best results dietary changes directed at improving sleep should be followed for several months.

Herbal medicines

- **Name of treatment and category:** _Ginkgo biloba_, _Hypericum perforatum_ (St. John's wort), _Panax ginseng_ (Ginseng), _Eschscholzia californica_ (California poppy), _Melissa officinalis_ (lemon balm) and _Withania somnifera_ (Ashwagondha) are herbals widely used in different healing traditions to treat insomnia and other medical and mental health problems.

- **How the treatment works:** Herbal medicines used to treat insomnia affect the levels of several neurotransmitters in the brain including serotonin, acetylcholine, GABA and others. In addition to _V. officinalis_ (reviewed in tier B), several other herbals are widely used to treat insomnia, however these herbals are supported by relatively less evidence. Extracts of the herbals *G. biloba* and *W. somnifera* may enhance sleep quality and may also improve cognitive functioning in individuals diagnosed with mild dementia. *H. perforatum*, widely used to treat depressed mood, may improve overall sleep quality. Some research findings suggest that taking a standardized preparation of *P. ginseng* improves sleep quality and increases daytime alertness.

- **Dosages (for natural products) or frequency of use (for whole body, mind-body or energy approaches):** Appropriate dosages of herbals used to treat insomnia vary with respect to age, the severity of insomnia and other factors.

- **Examples of safe and effective treatment combinations:** *Ginkgo biloba* may be safely combined with sedating antidepressants to improve sleep quality. One study reported that a combined regimen consisting of the extracts of California poppy, passionflower and lemon balm, together with vitamin B6 and melatonin resulted in significant and sustained improvement in sleep quality and duration in the absence of serious adverse effects.

- **Comments about adverse effects and warnings pertaining to treatment combinations that may result in potentially unsafe interactions and should be avoided:** Most herbals are safe when used following suggested dosing guidelines. *H. perforatum* may cause dizziness, irritability, rash, headache and dizziness. *P. ginseng* may cause agitation, diarrhea, headache and nervousness. *G. biloba* may cause upset stomach, headaches or dizziness. ***Caution: G. biloba increases bleeding time and should be discontinued at least 2 weeks before surgery.*** ***Warning: G. biloba should not be taken in combination with aspirin, warfarin or*** *other drugs or natural products that interfere with bleeding. Warning: H. perforatum and P. ginseng interact with select medications potentially resulting in serious toxicities.*

- **Average duration of treatment needed to achieve beneficial results:** Some individuals who take St. John's wort, *Ginkgo biloba* or *W. somnifera* on a regular daily basis for several weeks experience consistent improvements in sleep quality and duration.

Homeopathy

- **Name of treatment and category:** Homeopathy does not belong to a discrete category but may best fit in the category of 'energy-information' approaches.

- **How the treatment works:** Homeopathy is highly controversial in the Western medical community however many physicians study homeopathy and use it together with conventional Western medicine. Homeopathic remedies are made by diluting substances with water to achieve extremely low concentrations that are typically undetectable using available empirical means. Some theorists argue that homeopathy may have beneficial effects at the level of quantum mechanics. The homoepathic practitioner first determines the energetic constitution of each unique individual, then identifies the appropriate remedy aimed at correcting any energetic imbalances.

- **Dosages (for natural supplements) or frequency of use (for whole body, mind-body or energy approaches):** Few placebo-controlled studies have been done investigating homeopathic remedies for insomnia. In one small study individuals who received individualized homeopathic preparations for chronic insomnia experienced significant improvements in sleep quality and duration. It is important to comment that a variety of homeopathic remedies were used in that study.

- **Examples of safe and effective treatment combinations:** As homeopathic remedies probably contain no 'active' ingredients they may be safely combined with conventional or CAM approaches.

- **Comments about adverse effects and warnings pertaining to treatment combinations that may result in potentially unsafe interactions and should be avoided:** none reported

- **Average duration of treatment needed to achieve beneficial results:** In the study mentioned above, no individuals with chronic insomnia treated with individualized homeopathic preparations over a 3-month period experienced significant and sustained improvements in sleep quality and duration.

Lucid dreaming training

- **Name of treatment and category:** Lucid dreaming is a unique state of consciousness in which an individual is actually awake or self-aware while dreaming and able to change or control dream content. Training in lucid dreaming combines psychological and mind-body approaches.

- **How the treatment works:** Training in lucid dreaming can improve chronic insomnia caused by recurring disturbing dreams or nightmares. Various techniques permit the dreamer to confront disturbing dreams and change their content resulting in improved sleep. Lucid dreaming techniques such as *dialoging with* or *physically embracing* dream characters may reduce feelings of helplessness and terror as the individual learns that he or she can control frightening images or experiences. The use of word-association games and machines that use flashing lights or sounds to signal the sleeping brain during dreaming increase one's ability to become lucid. Training in lucid dreaming may reduce the severity and frequency of nightmares in individuals diagnosed with post-traumatic stress disorder (PTSD) which is often associated with chronic insomnia.

- **Dosages (for natural supplements) or frequency of use (for whole body, mind-body or energy approaches):** Training in lucid dreaming methods typically involves 4 to 6 weeks of daily dream journaling and weekly therapy sessions for practicing specific lucid dream-induction techniques focusing on insights related to recurrent nightmares.

- **Examples of safe and effective treatment combinations:** Training in lucid dreaming methods may be safely combined with other approaches.

- **Comments about adverse effects and warnings pertaining to treatment combinations that may result in potentially unsafe interactions and should be avoided:** none

- **Average duration of treatment needed to achieve beneficial results:** Some individuals who participate in a 4 to 6-week program in lucid dreaming training (above) are able to achieve lucidity and consistently reduce the frequency and intensity of recurring nightmares and reduce the frequency of middle waking, thereby improving sleep quality.

Passive body heating

- **Name of treatment and category:** Passive body heating is a whole-body approach.

- **How the treatment works:** Passive body heating increases the core body temperature which changes brain electrical activity resulting in general beneficial effects on the sleep-wake cycle in individuals with chronic insomnia.

- **Dosages (for natural supplements) or frequency of use (for whole body, mind-body or energy approaches):** Increasing the core body temperature to between 40 to 43 degrees centigrade by taking an immersion bath in hot water or a sauna for 10 to 30 minutes soon before bedtime makes it easier to fall asleep and improves sleep quality. ***NOTE: taking a hot bath earlier in the day has no effect on sleep.***

- **Examples of safe and effective treatment combinations:** Taking a hot bath or sauna may be safely used in combination with other approaches.

- **Comments about adverse effects and warnings pertaining to treatment combinations that may result in potentially unsafe interactions and should be avoided:** Taking a hot bath or sauna is generally safe. ***Caution: elderly and physically impaired individuals should be closely monitored when taking a hot bath or using a sauna to ensure their safety.***

- **Average duration of treatment needed to achieve beneficial results:** The beneficial effects of increasing core body temperature on sleep are almost immediate. Taking a hot bath (or sauna) on a nightly basis may result in sustained improvements in sleep in individuals with chronic insomnia.

Relaxation techniques

- **Name of treatment and category:** Relaxation techniques such as deep breathing, progressive muscle relaxation and guided imagery combine features of whole body and mind-body approaches.

- **How the treatment works:** Relaxation decreases the general excitability of the nervous system making it easier to fall asleep. Listening to soothing guided imagery soon before bedtime improves sleep quality. Guided imagery improves sleep quality in chronically anxious individuals. Progressive muscle relaxation involves tensing and relaxing muscle groups in different parts of the body producing feelings of calmness and mild sedation. Progressive muscle relaxation may help some individuals with insomnia fall asleep more easily.

- **Dosages (for natural supplements) or frequency of use (for whole body, mind-body or energy approaches):** Practicing simple relaxation techniques for 10 to 30 minutes soon before bedtime may increase the quality and duration of sleep.

- **Examples of safe and effective treatment combinations:** Relaxation techniques may be safely used in combination with prescription sleep aids in some cases improving their effectiveness. Practicing relaxation when using a prescription sleep aid is more effective than either approach alone.

- **Comments about adverse effects and warnings pertaining to treatment combinations that may result in potentially unsafe interactions and should be avoided:** none

- **Average duration of treatment needed to achieve beneficial results:** Some individuals with chronic insomnia experience significant improvements in sleep quality and duration following several weeks of regular relaxation practice.

Yoga

- **Name of treatment and category:** Yoga is an integral healing approach that combines training in specific postures, breathing techniques and mindfulness.

- **How the treatment works:** There are many styles of yoga. The regular practice of yoga has beneficial calming effects on the brain, improves physical strength and agility, and enhances mental and emotional well-being. Different yoga styles and practices have beneficial effects on insomnia, generalized anxiety, depressed mood and other mental health problems.

- **Dosages (for natural supplements) or frequency of use (for whole body, mind-body or energy approaches):** Practicing yoga 30 to 45 minutes 1 to 5 times weekly improves general sleep quality in individuals diagnosed with chronic insomnia.

- **Examples of safe and effective treatment combinations:** Yoga may be safely combined with other approaches. Some individuals who engage in a regular yoga practice are able to reduce their doses of prescription sleep medications without worsening symptoms of insomnia.

- **Comments about adverse effects and warnings pertaining to treatment combinations that may result in potentially unsafe interactions and should be avoided:** Gentle yoga practice carries little or no risk of injury. Individuals who have physical impairments or a chronic pain condition should consult with a physician or other qualified healthcare provider before starting a rigorous yoga practice.

- **Average duration of treatment needed to achieve beneficial results:** Many individuals with chronic insomnia experience sustained improvements in sleep quality and duration after practicing yoga 4 weeks or longer.

Before starting treatment

The treatment or treatment combination you decide to try after reading this book will be based on your unique history, symptoms, preferences and circumstances. As you learn how to think about your mental health care in a more holistic way using the information and methods in this book you will discover more effective approaches for taking care of your sleep problem.

Before starting one or more of the above treatments I encourage you to finish reading this entire book to make sure you know how to develop a plan that is *right for you*. If you have another mental health problem in addition to insomnia, I encourage you to read the book in the series on that condition or find another reliable source of information before starting any new treatment.

Deciding on a treatment plan that is *right for you*

General considerations

Now that you've learned about a variety of alternative treatment choices the next step is to decide on treatments that address your particular symptoms of insomnia keeping in mind treatment choices that are available where you live and within your budget.

As I mentioned earlier, because your symptoms are unique the best treatment plan for you may be different from the best treatment plan someone else. In other words, *there is no single best treatment for everyone who has insomnia*. I've created a simple method that will help you put together a treatment plan addressing your sleep problem.

The most appropriate treatment plan *for you* is based on:

- research evidence
- your response to treatments *you've* already tried
- your personal preferences
- treatments that are available where you live

- what you can afford

Do you have a medical problem that may be causing insomnia or interfering with response to treatment?

At the beginning of this book I described some medical problems that can cause or worsen insomnia, such as chronic pain, sleep apnea, diabetes, lung diseases, thyroid disease, dementia and neurological disorders. When an underlying medical problem is properly treated, sleep quality and duration may improve rapidly, and the treatment you've been taking without benefit may start to work better.

First steps

This section will guide you through the steps needed to develop a treatment plan that is appropriate for you whether you have mild, moderate or severe insomnia. The first step in deciding on an appropriate treatment plan involves identifying one or more treatments that you are *open to* trying.

When deciding on a treatment plan you probably have a better chance of *sleeping consistently better* if you use at least one tier A treatment. At the time of writing, tier A treatments of insomnia are bright light exposure (especially for sleep problems related to jet lag or shift work), EEG biofeedback training, and Valerian root extract. If you have severe chronic insomnia that is impairing your ability to function at work, in school or in other contexts you may need *to take a medication alone or with a tier A* treatment in order to sleep consistently better.

Even if you need to take a medication, you may benefit from taking one or more natural supplements or using other approaches described in this book. Natural supplements such as the herbals *Ginkgo biloba* (Ginkgo), *Hypericum perforatum* (St. Johns wort), *Panax ginseng* (Ginseng), and *Withania somnifera* (Ashwagandha), as well as melatonin, and the amino acids 5-HTP, L-tryptophan, are sometimes beneficial for severe insomnia and may be safely combined with antidepressants in some cases increasing their effectiveness. Besides natural supplements, other alternative approaches that are sometimes beneficial for severe insomnia include regular exercise, bright light exposure therapy, yoga and acupuncture.

If you are already taking a medication for insomnia, I strongly encourage you to *seek professional advice from a physician or other healthcare provider before starting any new treatment.*

Deciding on a treatment plan that is *right for you*

Since you've gotten this far, I am assuming that your sleep problem *isn't severe* enough to require an emergency room visit or hospitalization to evaluate possible underlying medical causes of insomnia. I am also assuming that *if a medical problem has been causing your insomnia, it has been evaluated and treated.* Finally, I am assuming that if you have been recently hospitalized for evaluation and treatment of a psychiatric disorder that is impairing your sleep (e.g., bipolar disorder or a psychotic disorder), that you've been discharged from the hospital and you are now feeling, functioning and sleeping better.

If these things describe your situation, you're ready to start working on a holistic treatment plan that addresses your sleep problem keeping in mind treatments that are available where you live, and affordable. On the other hand, if you have a severe sleep problem or think you have a medical problem that is interfering with your ability to sleep, I encourage you to find professional psychiatric or medical care before starting any new treatment including those discussed in this book.

Taking care of mild and moderately severe insomnia

If you have chronic mild or moderately severe insomnia, you may benefit from changes in diet and regular exercise. In addition to these lifestyle changes, certain natural supplements and yoga can help improve your sleep. Even if you have already tried some tier A approaches without success, you may benefit from a tier B or tier C approach. For example, tier B treatments such as acupuncture, cranioelectrotherapy stimulation (CES), melatonin, and listening to relaxing music at bedtime may help you sleep consistently better and reduce the dose of a prescription sleep aid, and possibly even discontinue it.

Before trying a Tier B treatment or a combination of treatments from Tier A and Tier B, I encourage you to first carefully review the detailed descriptions of Tier A treatments you've already tried to be sure you've used them in ways that *would be expected to be effective*. Some people who have used a particular natural supplement with disappointing results learn afterwards that they had been taking a dosage that was too low, stopped taking it before it had enough time to work, or were not using a quality brand. I encourage you to check the on-line resources at the end of this book to compare different brands of the natural supplement you've already tried. This will help you find out whether the supplement you previously used was a reputable brand.

If it turns out you didn't take a Tier A treatment at the recommended dosage or you used a brand of uncertain quality, I encourage you to try the same treatment again, this time taking a quality brand at the recommended dosage and for the recommended duration.

The above reasoning applies equally to treatments other than natural supplements. For example, if you previously tried yoga or another mind-body therapy, acupuncture or another therapy, and your response was disappointing I encourage you to check the information in the treatment summaries before concluding that the mind-body, whole body or energy treatment you previously tried is ineffective.

If you were not working with a skilled practitioner or trainer when you previously tried yoga or another mind-body approach, you *may not have used the most effective technique or practiced the approach for an amount of time that would be expected to consistently improve your sleep.* I encourage you to first re-

evaluate the way you previously practiced yoga (or another mind-body practice) to find out whether you were doing so in a way and for an amount of time that would be expected to improve sleep.

Other considerations

In addition to treatment preferences you have after reading this book, I encourage you to remain open to other approaches before deciding on a final treatment plan. If you've already tried several different approaches one at a time, you may have more success trying two or more approaches at the same time starting with treatments in Tiers A and B. This strategy can be especially helpful if:

- you've already tried most of the treatments listed in Tier A and they haven't lessened the severity of your insomnia
- a Tier A treatment you've previously tried helped you sleep better but caused side effects and you had to stop using it

- There is evidence that combining a particular Tier B or C treatment with a particular Tier A treatment will work better than taking a Tier A treatment alone

- a preferred Tier A treatment is unavailable where you live or too expensive

When to self-treat insomnia and when to seek advice from a healthcare provider

After you have identified treatment approaches you would like to try, the next step involves deciding whether to follow your treatment plan on your own or see a healthcare provider for expert advice and guidance. The information included under the various approaches will help you decide between self-care and working with a healthcare provider. I encourage you to consult with a physician or other health care provider if you have severe insomnia, or *if you are considering taking any natural supplement together with a medication.*

Below I've listed some important points that will help you find an experienced alternative healthcare practitioner of an approach that interests you:

- A physician or other conventional health care provider you already know may be able to help you find an experienced practitioner of an alternative therapy that interests you. You can probably get helpful information about local alternative medical practitioners from a clinic near you. Many alternative healthcare practitioners are members of a professional association of certified practitioners in their field. A representative of the appropriate professional association—whether it is on Chinese medicine, herbal medicine, yoga, or any another healing discipline—can probably recommend one or more practitioners near you.

- Once you've identified an experienced alternative practitioner, I encourage you to learn everything you can about their background, including education, training, licensing, and advanced certifications. Different professional groups and different countries impose a wide variety of requirements on health care providers in terms of training and standards of practice. The most important thing is to identify a practitioner who has a has a good reputation among his or her colleagues and extensive experience working with sleep disorders.

- The next step involves finding out what the treatment costs. I am assuming that many readers have health insurance that covers at least part of the cost of treatment. Not checking on cost and insurance issues before starting treatment can result in an expensive and brief encounter with even the most qualified practitioner, and leave you feeling disappointed and frustrated with fewer resources remaining to help you get the care you need.

- At the first session it is important to provide your new health care provider with a complete list of treatments you've already tried for insomnia including those that did *not work* or caused side effects. Your new provider will use this information to identify approaches that are more likely to be helpful while minimizing the risk of side effects.

- Be sure to tell your new health care provider *and all your providers*, about changes in your sleep problems, any new medical problems, and new treatments that you decide to try. Good communication between yourself and your health care providers will ensure they have the information they need to give you the best possible care.

Safety is *always* the *Number 1* priority

Safety is the *single most important consideration* when you are thinking about starting any new treatment—including a medication, a natural supplement—or a combination of two or more treatments.

Though serious safety problems are uncommon, combinations of certain supplements and medications can result in toxic interactions that may be dangerous and in rare cases life-threatening. I've included important safety information under all supplements so that you can review this material before starting a supplement or taking it with another supplement or a medication.

There is a great deal to know about safety that I cannot adequately cover in this short book. *Before taking any natural supplement together with a medication I encourage you to check the on-line resources at the end of this book to find out whether the specific combination you are considering is both effective and safe.*

Making changes along the way: re-evaluating your treatment plan and making it better

This section will help you find out how well your treatment plan is working and know what to do if it is not helping. You will learn when to continue your current treatment plan, change it, or stop it all together.

If you are not sleeping better *after following your initial treatment plan for the suggested amount of time* it is important re-evaluate what you are doing and consider making changes. If you have a medical problem that may be causing insomnia, I encourage you to see a physician or other health care provider to find out whether your medical problem requires treatment and to make sure it is not making your sleep problem worse or interfering with the beneficial effects of treatment.

If your treatment plan involves taking a natural supplement or using another approach reviewed in this book, and you've followed your plan for the *amount of time that is usually needed to achieve beneficial results but your sleep problem has not improved*, it is reasonable to consider:

- Increasing the dosage of a natural supplement or medication

- Finding a higher quality brand of a natural supplement or medication

- Increasing the frequency of yoga sessions or another mind-body practice you are pursuing

- Adding another approach to your existing treatment plan

- Switching to an entirely new treatment plan

- Stopping treatment all together

If you've already tried several approaches in tiers A and B but with limited success, you may benefit from combining a tier A and tier B treatment, two tier A treatments, or two treatments from tier B—*assuming it is safe to do so.*

Although tier C treatments are supported by less evidence than tier A and B treatments, some people benefit from tier C treatments. New research findings are constantly being reported at conferences and in medical journals showing that some treatments supported by weak or inconclusive research findings in the journal literature may actually be *more effective* than previously believed.

The amount of time it takes to sleep consistently better after starting any treatment or treatment combination, depends on many factors including how severe your sleep problem is, the particular treatment or treatments you are using, the amount of stress you are under, your general state of health and how closely you've been following your plan.

Most medications and supplements take time to work so it may take several weeks to sleep consistently better after starting a medication or a natural supplement. Information on how much time it usually takes for particular treatments to work is included in the treatment summaries.

Deciding when to change your treatment plan

The following questions will help you decide when to change your treatment plan.

How do I know if my current treatment plan is working?

If you are sleeping better most of the time your current treatment plan is probably working well. On the other hand, if your sleep problem is about the same as it was before you started treatment, your current treatment plan clearly isn't working, or you may not be using a particular treatment in the most effective way. Some people take longer than others to respond to the same dose of a specific medication, a natural supplement or the same level of commitment to yoga or another mind-body practice.

If your current treatment plan is helping you to sleep better some of the time but you continue to struggle with insomnia, you may benefit from adjusting dosages (of a medication or natural supplement) or increasing the frequency of workouts, a yoga practice, or another approach you've been trying, while continuing to follow the same general treatment plan as before. It is important to make any decisions about changing or stopping your treatment plan based on an accurate assessment of your symptoms. For this reason I encourage you to answer the questions in the same self-assessment inventory you used when deciding on your initial treatment plan. The results will help you to find out whether your sleep problem is the same, worse or better than before.

Taking inventory of your symptoms of insomnia will give you the information you need to decide whether to continue your current treatment plan, try something new, or stop treatment all together. Keeping a record of your answers will provide useful information about changes in your sleep problem over time and which treatments are more effective.

If I'm not sleeping consistently better how much longer should I wait before considering starting a new treatment?

The answer to this question depends on many factors that are different for each person. The amount of time needed to achieve consistent improvement in sleep in response to a specific treatment is listed under that treatment (i.e., when known). In general, if a treatment you are currently using worked in the past it will probably be effective this time. Unless you have severe insomnia that is impairing your ability to work, study or function in other ways, or you are experiencing serious side effects to a medication or natural supplement, I encourage you to continue your current treatment plan for several more weeks before trying something new.

How concerned should I be about side effects and what can I do if I get them? Making decisions about changing your treatment plan based on side effects has to do with how serious they are and how much they interfere with your ability to function. If you have mild side effects caused by a medication or a natural supplement that don't impair your ability to work, go to school, or interfere with other aspects of your life, your body may *get used* to these side effects fairly soon. On the other hand, if you are having side effects that interfere with your ability to function (e.g. sexual side effects, weight gain, problems with memory or concentration), it is prudent to stop your current treatment and try something new.

Depending on the medication or natural supplement that is causing side effects, changing the dosage or adding another medication or supplement can sometimes reduce or eliminate the problem. Of course, adding another medication or natural supplement *may also cause new side effects*. Before making any changes in your treatment plan aimed at reducing side effects, I encourage you to first get expert advice from a physician or other health care provider.

When should I try something new in addition to my current treatment? How do I decide what to try next?

As a general rule it is best to keep your treatment plan as simple as possible and avoid particular combinations of treatments that cause potentially serious safety problems. If you are sleeping better on your current treatment plan and your sleep problem isn't severe, I encourage you to wait a little longer before trying something new. On the other hand, if you aren't sleeping consistently better most of the time on your current treatment, or have severe insomnia, or a serious mental health problem like depression or bipolar disorder, it is prudent to consider trying something new that may enhance the beneficial effects of your current treatment.

Deciding whether to add a new treatment to your current treatment plan depends on the *likelihood that the change will result in improvement in sleep that would otherwise not take place*. Deciding whether to add another treatment to your current plan also depends on *whether the potential risk of side effects outweighs the potential benefits of starting a new treatment.*

Before deciding whether to try two or more approaches at the same time I encourage you to first review the information in the treatment summaries to learn about specific combinations known to be effective and safe. In order to minimize the risk of side effects and potentially unsafe interactions please exercise caution when adding any new treatment to an existing treatment— whether it is a medication, a natural supplement or something else.

When should I stop what I'm taking and try something new or take no treatment at all?

If you are taking a quality brand natural product or medication at the recommended dosage, or using in a whole body, mind-body or energy therapy on a regular basis but you are not sleeping consistently better, it may be time to discontinue your current treatment plan and wait before starting any new treatment. In this case, if you are taking a medication or a natural supplement under the advice of a physician or alternative medical practitioner, I encourage you to see your healthcare provider for advice on how to safely discontinue the medication (or supplement) before starting any new treatment. For the most part, gradually decreasing the dosage of a medication or supplement reduces the risk of side effects that can take place when abruptly stopping treatment. In some cases, especially for mild or moderately severe insomnia, you may sleep better after stopping a medication or a natural supplement.

By maintaining a healthy lifestyle including regular exercise, engaging in a regular mind-body practice, and maintaining a healthy diet, mild and moderately severe insomnia may improve even in the absence of treatment. However, if you are impaired by severe chronic insomnia, it is prudent to consider adding another treatment to boost the effectiveness of your current treatment, or to consider switching to an entirely new treatment. Before doing either of the above, I encourage you to first consult with a physician or other healthcare provider experienced in managing insomnia for expert advice and guidance. When deciding whether to try any new treatment for insomnia use the same steps you followed when developing your initial treatment plan. Remember, deciding on a treatment plan always starts with answering questions about your symptoms, and finding out whether a medical problem is causing your symptoms or interfering with your response to treatment.

When should I see a healthcare provider for expert advice including questions about dosages, concerns about adverse effects, or to find out whether I have a medical problem?

It is prudent to consult with a physician or another health care provider if you have side effects caused by a medication or a natural supplement. I strongly encourage you to see a healthcare provider if you have or *think you have* a medical problem in order to get a thorough evaluation and to find out whether a medical problem is causing your sleep problem, making it worse or interfering with response to treatment.

Repeating the steps until you find a treatment plan that *works* for you

Sometimes it is necessary to try many different approaches in order to get to a treatment plan that works. Every time you go through the process of deciding on a treatment plan you will have a better understanding of your sleep problem and how it changes over time. You will also have useful insights about treatments that work as well as ones that *don't work*. When evaluating your sleep problem, you can use the same self-assessment questionnaire as many times as you need to. By saving your answers you can track how your sleep problem responds to changes in your treatment plan. This information will help you decide whether to continue your current treatment, try something new or stop treatment all together.

If you have not experienced consistent improvement in the quality and duration of sleep after trying two different treatment plans, I encourage you to seek advice from a health care provider. *Finally—and I can't emphasize this point strongly enough—if you are severely depressed or have another serious mental health problem, or if you think you have a medical problem that may be causing insomnia or making it worse, I encourage you to seek immediate medical care.*

Summary of main points

Below I summarize the most important points in this book including key steps involved in developing a safe, effective and affordable treatment plan based on your history, symptoms, preferences and circumstances:

- **If in addition to insomnia, you are severely depressed or if you have another serious mental health problem that is impairing your ability to function, I urge you to *seek urgent care at the nearest hospital or emergency room.***

- This book is offered as a practical resource on the safe and effective *alternative* treatments of insomnia.

- Alternative medicine sometimes called 'complementary and alternative medicine or CAM—consists of approaches that are currently not used in mainstream Western medicine (also called 'biomedicine' and 'allopathic medicine').

- Integrative medicine is a person-centered approach to care that incorporates mainstream Western medical treatments and CAM approaches.

- Integrative mental health care is the area of integrative medicine aimed at optimizing emotional and mental wellness and treating specific mental health problems.

- If you've recently been hospitalized or evaluated in an emergency room for severe insomnia or a serious mental health or medical problem and you are now sleeping and functioning better, this book will help you find reliable information about alternative treatment approaches.

- If you *have* a medical problem that has not been diagnosed, is not being treated, or has recently been getting worse, I encourage you to see a physician or other healthcare provider before making *any* changes in your current treatment plan for insomnia or starting any new treatment.

Medical problems that can cause or worsen insomnia include sleep apnea, diabetes, lung diseases, thyroid disease, dementia and neurological disorders. Many medications can interfere with normal sleep. Impaired sleep frequently occurs together with severe depressed mood, bipolar mania and other serious mental health problems.

- The first step in developing a treatment plan that is right for you involves taking inventory of your insomnia symptoms using the self-assessment questionnaires provided on the companion website. Your answers will help you better understand the nature and severity of your sleep problem.

- After taking inventory the next step is to carefully review the evidence for various treatments and to identify those treatments that make sense for you.

- The next step involves deciding whether to start treatment on your own or to work with a healthcare provider.

- Mild or moderately severe symptoms of insomnia often respond to changes in lifestyle such as stress management, improved nutrition and more frequent exercise.

- Severe or chronic insomnia seldom responds to lifestyle changes alone, and may require long-term treatment with a prescription medication, a natural supplement or a medication and natural supplement in combination. Decisions about combining two or more medications or supplements should always be based on scientific evidence and safety considerations. *If you have severe or chronic insomnia, I strongly encourage you work closely with a physician or other health care provider who can evaluate you and advise you on a treatment plan that is appropriate for you.*

- Even if you need a medication or a natural supplement in order to sleep consistently better, making positive lifestyle changes such as exercising more often, good nutrition, and a stress reduction program, can significantly improve your sleep quality.

- When deciding on a treatment plan first consider tier A treatments supported by strong evidence. If you have already tried several tier A treatments without benefit, I encourage you to review the detailed information in this book on those treatments to make sure you previously used a quality brand (i.e. if it is a natural supplement) at the recommended dosage and for the recommended period of time. If you've already tried exercise, yoga or another mind-body approach, or an energetic approach (e.g., EEG biofeedback, cranio-electrotherapy stimulation and acupuncture), but were disappointed in the results, I encourage you to review the information on that particular approach to make sure you used it in a way and for a period of time that would be expected to help you sleep consistently better.

- If you discover that you did not try a tier A treatment at the optimal dosage and duration, I encourage you to try that treatment again. This time make sure you use the recommended dosage of a quality brand for the recommended amount of time. If you previously tried a mind-body or energetic approach that is known to be beneficial for insomnia, but without success, I encourage you try that approach again, this time closely following recommendations on frequency and duration of treatment that would most likely achieve beneficial results.

- An important consideration is deciding whether to try one treatment or a combination or two or more treatments at the same time. *Examples of beneficial combinations as well as unsafe combinations to be avoided* are included in the detailed descriptions under the various treatments.

- If you are not sleeping consistently better *after following the initial treatment plan for the recommended amount of time,* I encourage you to find a health care provider to obtain diagnostic tests in order to make sure that a medical problem is not causing insomnia, making your sleep problem worse, or interfering with your response to treatment.

- If your sleep problem does not improve consistently after you've followed your treatment plan for a period after which you should expect beneficial results, I encourage you to consider switching to a different treatment, preferably one that belongs to tier A or tier B. Where known, the amount of time in which you should expect improvement in response to a particular treatment is discussed under each treatment. Depending on the severity of your sleep problem, it may be helpful to continue your current treatment while adding one or more new approaches.

- Make sure you know about safety concerns associated with any treatment or treatment combinations you are considering. Safety problems are described under the specific treatments. *Before combining two or more treatments first review the comments on safe and effective treatment combinations as well as warnings pertaining to particular treatment combinations. It is always best to avoid combining two or more treatments that can potentially result in a toxic interaction.* If you decide to combine two or more treatments after reviewing the information in this book, I encourage you to first consult with a health care provider for expert advice and guidance.

- From time to time it is important to take a close look at your sleep problem—*even when your treatment plan is working well.* Doing a self-inventory by answering standardized questions will help you understand your sleep problem better and determine whether you are experiencing significant new symptoms of insomnia or another mental health problem such as depression, anxiety or bipolar disorder that may be interfering with normal sleep.

- Continue to modify your treatment plan on an on-going basis using an appropriate self-assessment inventory to document any changes in sleep. Changes in your sleep pattern over time may call for changes in the treatment plan. If you are not sleeping consistently better after trying at least two different treatment plans for the recommended period please seek professional care for formal evaluation and expert advice.

- If you are still experiencing mild or moderately severe insomnia after trying at least two separate treatment plans, you may be able to sleep just as well even after discontinuing treatment. Many people with mild or moderately severe insomnia benefit a great deal from lifestyle changes including regular exercise, improved nutrition, and stress management.

Going deeper

After reading this e-book on integrative management of insomnia you may want to learn more. You can find in-depth information in my other books:

- *An Integrative Paradigm for Mental Health Care: Ideas and Methods Shaping the Future*, Springer, 2019

- *Textbook of Integrative Mental Health Care*, Thieme Medical, 2006

- *Integrative Mental Health Care: A Therapist's Handbook*, Norton 2009

- *Complementary and Alternative Treatments in Mental Health Care*, American Psychiatric Association, Inc. 2006

- *Chinese Medical Psychiatry: A Textbook and Clinical Manual*, Blue Poppy Press, 2000

You can find links to all of my books, as well as many full-text articles and conference presentations on my website http://progressivepsychiatry.com/

Finding quality products and services on the Internet

After you've decided on the treatment plan that makes sense for you the next step is to find quality products and services that you can use. This section includes valuable internet resources that will help you select safe, effective and affordable products and services. Some of the resources listed are free while others charge a subscription fee.

General resources on complementary and alternative treatment approaches

- **Progressive Psychiatry** http://progressivepsychiatry.com/ This is the author's website. It includes a comprehensive list of on-line resources on both mainstream mental health care and complementary and alternative medicine (CAM) approaches. You can find several full-text articles published by Dr. Lake as well as presentations made at various conferences over the years. The site also includes a blog on integrative mental health care and links to all of Dr. Lake's books.

- **The National Center for Complementary and Integrative Health (NCCIH)** https://nccih.nih.gov is part of the National Institutes of Health (NIH). NCCIH is dedicated to exploring complementary and alternative healing practices in the context of rigorous science, training complementary and alternative medicine (CAM) researchers, and disseminating authoritative information to the public and professionals. The site contains extensive reviews of research on all non-medication treatment approaches. A citation index contains over 200,000 citations of studies on all areas of non-conventional medicine indexed in the National Library of Medicine beginning in 1966. The section includes valuable advice on how to find qualified practitioners of alternative and integrative medicine. The site includes information **en Español.**

Resources on dietary supplements (no fee)

- **National Institutes of Health Office of Dietary Supplements** https://ods.od.nih.gov/ provides an extensive on-line library of dietary supplement fact sheets for widely used herbals and other natural products. Different versions are available for consumers and health professionals. The site includes frequently asked questions (FAQs) and links to scientific monographs. The site includes some information **en Español.**

- **Medline Plus Supplement Information** https://medlineplus.gov/druginformation.html is a service of the U.S. National Library of Medicine, National Institutes of Health. It includes a comprehensive library of on-line monographs on prescription drugs as well as herbals and other natural product supplements. Each monograph includes safety information on adverse effects and interactions. The site also includes free mental health screening tools, educational brochures, videos and podcasts on common mental health problems.

- **Drugs.com** https://www.drugs.com/ includes a comprehensive library of on-line monographs on prescription medications and natural products including extensive information on adverse effects. It includes an on-line tool for checking interactions. Different versions are available for consumers and health professionals. The information on the site is also available **en Español**.

- **National Herbalists Association of Australia** https://www.nhaa.org.au Founded in 1920, the National Herbalists Association of Australia is the oldest natural therapies association in Australia, and the only national professional body of medical herbalists. Their mission is to serve and support membership (Medical Herbalists and Naturopaths) and to promote and protect the profession and practice of herbal medicine. This website is a portal to on-line resources covering all aspects of herbal medicine as well as complementary and alternative medicine in general. It includes links to valuable resources on research, nutrition, herbals and other natural product supplements, professional associations, educational resources, and reputable distributors and suppliers of herbals and other natural products.

- **The World Health Organization's (WHO) traditional medicine portal** https://www.who.int/traditional-complementary-integrative-medicine/en/ provides a traditional medicine fact sheet and links to worldwide health care resources. WHO seeks to promote international collaboration and cooperation in the study and use of traditional healing approaches in mental health care.

Resources on natural products and other non-medication treatments (fee)

- **ConsumerLab.com** https://www.consumerlab.com/

provides independent test results and information to help consumers and healthcare professionals evaluate health, wellness, and nutrition products. ConsumerLab is a certification company and enables companies of all sizes to have their products voluntarily tested for potential inclusion in its list of Approved Quality products and bear its seal of approval. The site is a valuable consumer resource for evaluating different natural products and brands and identifying brands that are both safe and effective.

- **Natural   Medicines** https://naturalmedicines.therapeuticresearch.com is a subscription service that provides valuable information on natural products and other non-medication approaches. Like Consumerlab.com, Natural Medicines provides independent reviews of supplements that are authoritative and easy to read. The site provides links to valuable databases on natural products and other approaches. It also includes consumer monographs, patient handouts and offers continuing education credit on different topics to health professionals.

- **Herb** **Research** **Foundation** http://www.herbs.org/hrfinfo.html includes expert compilations on specific herbals that contain carefully selected articles, studies, and discussions by experts that are available as downloads or in print form. The work of the Herb Research Foundation is based on its dedicated holdings of more than 300,000 scientific articles on thousands of herbs.

Made in the USA
Middletown, DE
11 January 2021